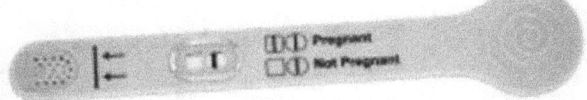

Fertility Hacks

Learn Old and New Tricks to Boost Your Fertility

Published By Shaharm Publications

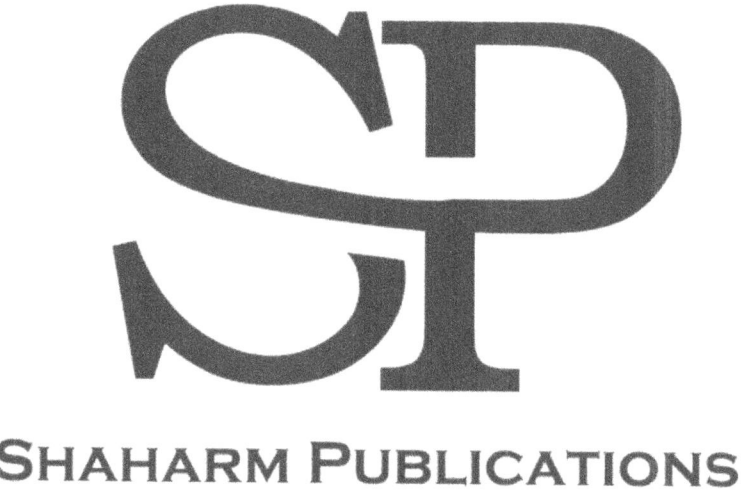

SHAHARM PUBLICATIONS

For a full list of books by Shaharm Publications,
please go to:

http://www.shaharmpublications.com

Table of Contents

1. So You Want to Have a Baby...   2

2. Why Consider These Fertility Options?   6

3. Fertility Advancement through the Ages   9

4. Have You Been Told That You Can't Have Children?   11

5. Taking a Look at the Monthly Cycle   14

6. For Him: Body Health and Sperm Health   17

7. For Her: the Importance of Diet and Exercise   21

8. For Her: Getting the Right Fluids   25

9. For Her: Acupuncture and Other Alternative Options   29

10. For Couples: Frequency and Timing of Intercourse   32

11. For Couples: Kick the Habit   36

12. For Couples: Staying Healthy Together   39

13. For Couples: Let Go of the Stress   41

14. For Couples: Is It Time to See a Doctor?   44

1. So You Want to Have a Baby...

The birth of a child is one of the most precious events that can happen for a couple. In fact, many individuals wait for years in order to be able to have children of their own. Unfortunately, there are also times when it is very difficult to become pregnant, and you may have even been told that you are unable to get pregnant. According to the statistics, there are 6.7 million women in the United States between the ages of 15-44 that have a difficulty becoming pregnant. Among women in the same age group that are married, 6% are considered to be infertile and some 7.4 million have used infertility services at some time in the past.

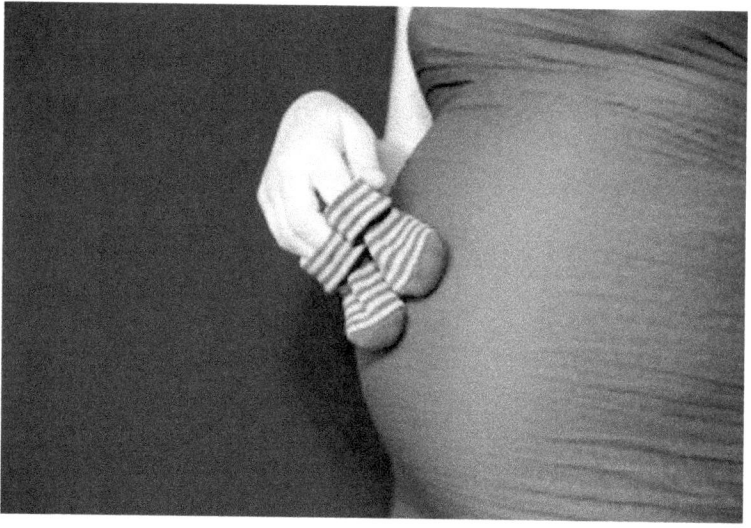

Although the numbers may seem to be grim on the surface, there are also many millions of couples that are able to successfully conceive, even those who were told in the past that they would have a difficulty with doing so. It is important for you to understand that you can get beyond this difficulty, and if you follow the advice that is available in this book, you certainly can increase the likelihood that you will have a child of your own.

The first thing that we will do is to consider the benefits of having children and using some sort of fertility hack to do so. In addition, we are going to take a look at some of the ways in which fertility was approached throughout the ages. That kind of discussion can be very interesting, not only because it shows you how far we've come with medical advances, but that things that worked thousands of years ago and were understood by the majority are still able to work today.

If you have been told that you can't have children, don't despair. There are plenty of instances of couples that were told that they were unable to conceive and now they have children and at times, even multiple children. Although medical science has advanced through the ages, it is still an imperfect science, which is probably why they are said to be "practicing" medicine. The bad news may be distressing, but it is not absolute.

The monthly cycle is perhaps one of the most important things to understand when it comes to getting pregnant. After all, women go through the cycle every month and there are certain times in which it is more likely for them to conceive. Of course, there are many factors that need to come in to play in order for things to go off successfully, but if you follow the cycle and understand how to do so properly, it can increase the possibility that you will become pregnant.

We will start off our discussion on different factors that can improve your chances of conceiving by talking about the male in the equation. There are a number of things that the man can do to improve the health, not only of his body but also of the sperm. Some of these are relatively easy to put into place, and it can make a difference, even making it possible for you to conceive when at one time, the man may have been considered infertile.

For the woman, we have several different suggestions as to how to improve your odds of conception. The first thing that we will discuss is diet and exercise, which certainly is important when it comes to the health of the body. Although eating a proper diet and getting some exercise is not going to magically make you fertile, it can go a long way in helping you to conceive. We will also talk about the necessity of drinking the proper fluids and enough of them. In addition, we will talk about some alternative treatment options, including acupuncture.

After discussing men and women separately, we are going to talk about a few different things that can be done as a couple in order to improve your odds of conception. One of the first things that we will discuss is the frequency and timing of intercourse. This is something that needs to be understood properly, because most people have it upside down when it comes to how frequently to have sex in order to conceive successfully. We will take a look at the truth behind the matter.

Do you smoke cigarettes or use tobacco of any kind? It doesn't matter if you are the man or the woman; the use of tobacco is going to hurt your odds of conception. Kicking the habit can be difficult but if you want to increase your chances of having a baby, it is important to do so. Of course, kicking the smoking habit is also going to be beneficial for the health of the baby, as well as for the health of the new parents.

It is also important for you to consider your overall health, including the types of foods that you are eating, how much fluid you are drinking and the exercise that you are getting every day. These things can be worked on separately but when you work on them as a couple, it can really make a difference in your ability to stick with the program for the long-term.

Do you have a lot of stress in your life? Stress is a problem for most people, and today, it is not out of the ordinary to have stress to the point where it is chronic. If you suffer from high levels of stress, letting go of the problem is one of the first steps that you need to take if you want to conceive successfully. We will talk about how stress affects the body and what you can do to reduce your stress levels quickly and easily.

Finally, we are going to talk about the possibility that you might benefit from seeing a doctor. Medical science has certainly helped many people to conceive and to carry the child through to delivery, when at one time, it may have been difficult for the couple to do so. Although there are a lot of natural options that are discussed in this publication, there may also be times when it is necessary for you to trust in medical science and what it has to offer.

The choice to bring a new life into the world is one that should not be taken lightly. It is not just a matter of conception, pregnancy and delivery; you are embarking on a long-term project that will have many ups and downs along the way. If you are able to have a child, you will find that it is one of the best choices that you ever made in life. It is our hope that this publication will assist you in conceiving a child successfully.

2. Why Consider These Fertility Options?

Throughout the pages of this publication, we are going to discuss many factors that allow you to conceive a child and to do so with success. You will find that many of the options available are natural and have many benefits associated with them, not only the conception and delivery of the child itself. In this chapter, we are going to consider some of those additional benefits. You will find that it provides you with motivation to embark on this journey that has something wonderful at the end of it.

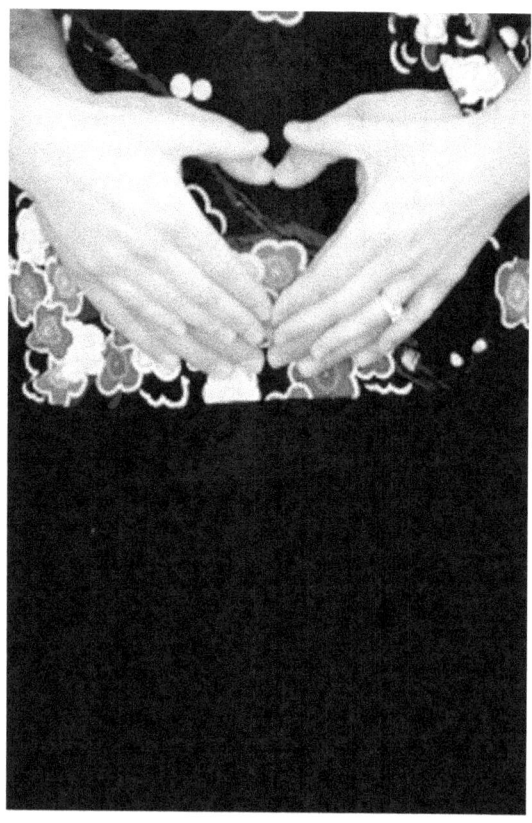

Physical Health - One of the recurring themes that you will discover in this publication is that you need to improve your overall health if you want to improve your possibilities of getting pregnant. Although it certainly can assist you in conceiving, eating a proper diet, getting plenty of sleep and doing some exercise on a regular basis is going to have many physical health benefits as well. You will no doubt appreciate those benefits very quickly.

Mental Health - Along with improving your physical health, it is likely that you are also going to see some mental health benefits by applying the suggestions in this publication as well. One of the ways that it may be seen is that you will feel better about yourself and about your lot in life when you are caring for yourself properly. In addition, improving the way that you eat can help to improve your mental health by removing dangerous chemicals from your diet, including sugar and many preservatives.

Closeness - Although much of this publication is about improving fertility for either the man or the woman, even when it is done as a couple, it is also done individually. As a result, there are additional benefits that may be experienced by both individuals in the relationship. As you continue to work together toward this common goal, you will find that you are drawing closer together and appreciating all that it has to offer.

Intimacy - Something that is lacking in many relationships is a degree of healthy intimacy. Obviously, when you're trying to conceive a child, it is necessary to be intimate with each other and you will appreciate the fact that you are able to share such closeness on a regular basis.

Knowledge - When you are trying to conceive a child and you are doing what is necessary to do it successfully, you will be working in many different areas of your life. Not only are you trying to improve your physical health, you're trying to improve your overall outlook, your stress levels and more. It is important to understand yourself and your body and when you are finished with this publication, you will walk away with a newfound appreciation for what you have available.

Although there are many different benefits that are associated with trying to conceive a child, those that were mentioned above are some that are experienced by most individuals in the relationship. There is no doubt that you will also experience other benefits, both alone and as you continue to work together as a couple.

3. Fertility Advancement through the Ages

Throughout the history of the human race, fertility and the ability to conceive a child has always been of importance. In fact, it was often of more importance to individuals during times past than it is to the general population today. After all, we have a good idea of what happens during conception, and we certainly have a far greater understanding than what our ancient ancestors had. It is interesting, however, to look at the history of what was believed about fertility, because it can give you an inside view as to what many people still believe today.

One of the more interesting things to consider about fertility is the fact that it often was part of the religious services in ancient times. Most cultures had some sort of fertility rites that were practiced, sometimes in a religious setting. In addition, there were often gods that were specific to fertility and if those gods were upset, it was thought it could affect the conception of children in that society.

Although the ancient fertility rites have all but disappeared, it is still a part of religion today in many instances. For example, some religions still have patron Saints for that very purpose and there may be prayers that are said for that reason as well. Although we understand it to be superstition today, it is still a carryover from those ancient times.

Those societies also had a lot of theories as to how a woman could more easily conceive a child. For example, in ancient Roman times, it was suggested that the possibility of a woman getting pregnant could be seen by her outward appearance. This would include the size of her eyes, if she had a large head or if her forehead was protruding. The ancient Romans also thought that the best time to conceive a child was immediately after menstruation ceased. It was also thought that the man and the woman should be fairly healthy and that they should be sober during the intimate act, especially woman. Unfortunately, it was also thought that an act of violence that occurred during conception would make the child more like the aggressor.

Medical science has also come a long way in how they handle fertility as well. Thousands of years ago, it was not uncommon in many cultures for bloodletting and other rituals to take place in an effort to increase the possibility that a couple would be able to conceive. Although many of these fertility rites were religious in nature, they were also done with the blessing of medical science as well.

In more recent years, medical science has turned to actual science in order to improve the possibility that the couple could conceive. Although it has been moving in this direction for many years, it was the first test tube baby, who was born on July 25, 1978 that really put it into the limelight. This leap forward in medical technology is now seen as commonplace, as in vitro fertilization and fertility drugs are readily available.

There has also been somewhat of a reversal as far as fertility options are concerned. Although medical doctors may be able to provide some opportunities for the conception of a child that were not available before, there are also many individuals that are looking to alternative methods and natural health to conceive a child. That is the primary information that is provided in this publication, although we will look into modern medical science and the possibility that it can assist you as well.

4. Have You Been Told That You Can't Have Children?

If you have been trying to conceive for quite some time and you have been unable to do so, you may have been told by a doctor or perhaps by someone you trust that you may not be able to have children. Although this is a common occurrence, and as we discussed previously, there are millions of women in the United States alone who are unable to conceive children, it is not an absolute problem. In this chapter, we will take a look at some of the possibilities and why you should never give up hope in being able to have a child.

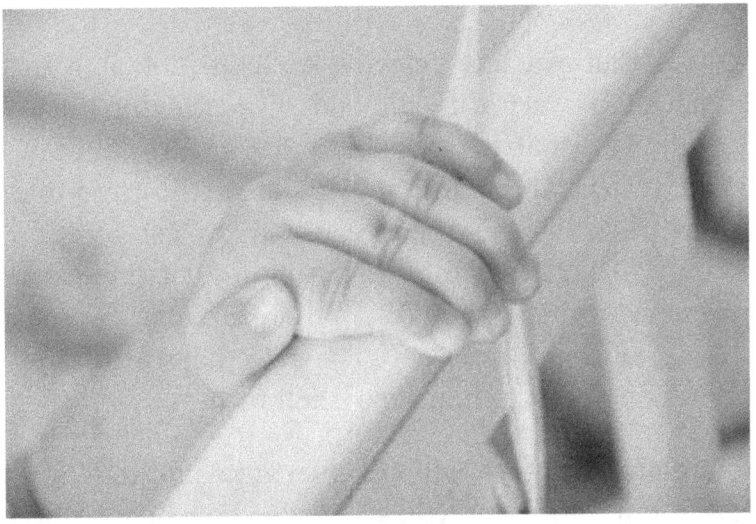

First of all, it's important to understand the definition of infertility as to how it may be understood by a physician that is giving you the bad news. According to the World Health Organization, infertility is a disease of the reproductive system defined as the failure to achieve a clinical pregnancy after 12 months or more of regular, unprotected sexual intercourse. It is important to note that the man in the relationship is the one that can be tested in a laboratory setting to determine if he is having a problem with infertility. The woman is often unable to make that determination, until enough time has passed that she could be termed as "clinically infertile".

It is also important to recognize that in some cases, the ability to conceive a child is not difficult but the possibility of carrying it to full term and delivering a healthy baby may be the problem. This publication is primarily geared toward those that are trying to conceive a child and may not have been able to do so in the past. Following the tips in this publication can also help women who are having difficulty carrying a child to term, as the improvement in your general health may assist in that regard.

Being told that you are infertile and are not able to have children can be very difficult and disheartening. It doesn't mean, however, that the possibility for having children does not exist. In fact, there are many women who were told that they were infertile and tried very hard to get pregnant for years, only to find that they were able to get pregnant after they "stopped trying". In addition, there are many women that were told that they would never be able to have children that now have one or more children of their own.

There are also different types of infertility and understanding those different types can help you to see how big of a problem it is for you.

Disability - When you have infertility as a result of a disability, it may affect your ability to conceive or carry a child to term permanently. In many countries, disability that affects infertility is common, as they may have had unsafe abortions or maternal sepsis. Worldwide, it is the fifth leading health problem of serious concern.

Primary - This type of infertility occurs when a woman is unable to successfully conceive a child or to carry the child to term and experience a live birth. There are many women who are considered to have a problem with primary infertility that eventually were able to have a child of their own.

Secondary - This type of infertility is very similar to primary infertility, but it occurs after a woman was able to conceive a child and have a live birth. If there is a difficulty with conception or carrying the baby to full term after a successful birth, it is considered a secondary infertility.

The bottom line is that if you have been told that you are unable to have children, it is still often possible to do so. By following the information that is available in this publication, you are increasing your odds of having a baby of your own.

5. Taking a Look at the Monthly Cycle

Although there is much to discuss about conceiving a child, it is important to start with the most basic information. As far as conception is concerned, it all has to do with the monthly cycle that every woman goes through. In this chapter, we are going to take a look at the menstrual cycle and to provide you with some basic information as to what can be done in order to improve your odds of conceiving by your newfound knowledge.

Although the length of the cycle is going to vary from one woman to another, it commonly is between 23 and 35 days in length. The first day of the menstrual cycle, however, is the first day that you have your period. For some women, this phase lasts for up to seven days but it is not uncommon for it to last only three days in some women. It is also during this time that the hormones fluctuate in the female body, so you may experience some mood swings and some menstrual pain. During your period, the lining of the womb is being shed.

Your body is also producing a hormone that is known as the follicle stimulating hormone (FSH) during this time. The pituitary gland, which is located in the brain, is responsible for producing that hormone. Each follicle within your ovary contains an immature egg and this hormone is what causes the body to develop the egg so that it is prepared for conception. Your levels of estrogen increase during this time as well.

Although FSH may affect many different follicles, one of them will likely become dominant during this time, and the egg will continue to develop within it. As your estrogen continues to increase, the womb is producing a new lining that includes blood along with various nutrients that will help to sustain the new life once the conception occurs. Estrogen also causes changes to occur in your cervical mucus, which makes it more likely for the sperm to be able to travel through it successfully.

As the estrogen continues to rise in the body, luteinizing hormone is produced and causes the egg from the dominant follicle to release. At this point, ovulation has occurred and the egg is now traveling through the fallopian tube on its way to the womb.

One of the more common misconceptions about ovulation is that it takes place on the 14th day after the start of the period. In reality, it varies from one woman to another, depending upon her own physical makeup and the timing of her menstrual cycle.

When the egg is released from the ovary, it begins its descent through the fallopian tube and it will typically be alive for approximately 24 hours after it has been released from the follicle. Male sperm, on the other hand, is able to live for up to five days so if it is already in the fallopian tubes, it is likely that it will meet the egg as it is on its journey.

After the egg is released, the production of estrogen starts to drop off and another hormone, known as progesterone, begins to be produced by the female body. The womb will react as a result of the progesterone and will produce a thicker lining in anticipation of the conceived egg dropping from the fallopian tubes. The production of progesterone, along with estrogen may cause some discomfort during this time that could include breast tenderness, depression, irritability and bloating.

If the egg that drops into the womb is not fertilized, the production of progesterone drops. Eventually, the lower levels of those hormones will cause the womb to begin to shed its lining once again, which occurs on the first day of the next menstrual cycle. It will then begin the cycle all over again, starting on day one.

6. For Him: Body Health and Sperm Health

If you have been to a fertility doctor, you likely have heard information as to whether the man or the woman is having difficulty with infertility. Although it may automatically be assumed that it is the fault of the woman, there are many times when it is the fault of man. In addition, it is not uncommon to be told that you are unable to have children and that it is not able to be determined why that is the case. Regardless of whether the man tested as infertile or not, however, the following can be done to help improve the fertility of the man and to increase your odds for conception.

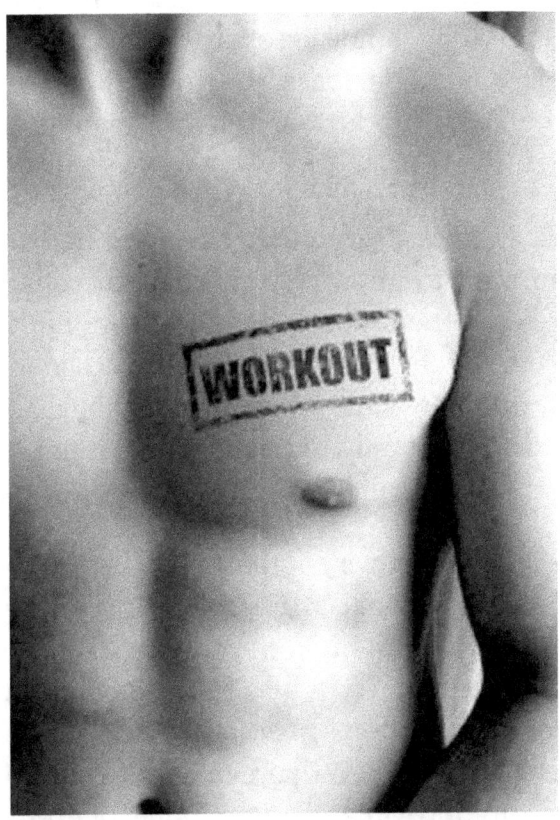

In this chapter, we are going to talk about some of the ways in which men can improve their ability to do their part in the conception process. You will find that it is not only a matter of improving sexual and sperm health; it is also a matter of improving your overall health as well. In that way, the benefits are going to extend far beyond the possibility of being able to conceive a child.

One important factor, and one that will be discussed further in another chapter of this publication, is the frequency with which you have intercourse. Most men will feel as if they should have intercourse every day in order to improve the odds conception. Although it certainly is statistically possible to improve your odds by doing so, it is not really necessary. The male sperm can last for up to five days after ejaculation, so having sex every day is not necessarily going to improve your odds. In fact, it may decrease your odds because your body may not be able to produce sperm fast enough to keep you fertile.

Typically, having sex every other day is going to be the best option if you want to improve your odds for conception. That gives your body the opportunity to keep up with sperm production effectively. It is also not a good idea for you to avoid sex in order to build up sperm. Although it may seem like a good idea, it actually increases the number of unhealthy sperm that you have available.

Staying healthy is also very important when it comes to the possibility of conceiving a child. Eating a healthy diet, including plenty of fruits and vegetables, is one of the best choices that you can make in life. You should also try to avoid any boxed or canned items, because they contain unhealthy preservatives and additives that can affect your sperm health as well. Aim for approximately 20 minutes of exercise per day, even if you have to split it between two or three sessions during the day.

Drinking is very important if you're trying to improve your health and the health of your sperm. Of course, I'm not talking about drinking alcohol, coffee or any other beverage other than clear, clean water. Many men tend to be dehydrated, and it is often a chronic condition that has been an issue throughout the majority of their lives. Drinking a minimum of eight glasses of water throughout the day is important if you want to improve your health. Try to avoid any sugary drinks, coffee, or drinking too much alcohol, as they can all have a negative impact on your health and your sperm count.

More than likely, you have heard the advice that you should switch to boxers if you want to improve your sperm count. Although this advice has been around for many years, and the science behind it is sound, it has been shown to be ineffective at improving sperm count and health. When you look at what is behind the suggestion, and that is keeping the testicles at a comfortable and controllable temperature, it can have an impact on your ability to conceive. Avoid hot tubs or sitting in hot water for an extended amount of time, as it can affect your sperm production significantly.

If you are exposed any type of pesticides or dangerous chemicals on a regular basis, this is something that may need to be controlled as well. Of course, it is important for you to do so for a variety of reasons but studies have shown that exposure to those kinds of chemicals can have a negative impact on your sperm health and production. If you don't avoid those chemicals for any other reason, do it for the health of your sperm.

Finally, one of the biggest problems that many men experience that can have an effect on their ability to have children is their stress level. This is something that we will discuss in detail in another chapter of this publication, but it was also important to mention it here. If you're constantly stressed out at work, at home or in any other location, take the necessary steps to reduce your stress levels. It can really make a difference.

7. For Her: the Importance of Diet and Exercise

In most parts of the world, we are dealing with an epidemic of obesity. This is a problem that has many obvious concerns behind it, but it is also a major player when it comes to infertility. More than likely, you have been told to lose some weight if you are obese, but the need to do so is compounded when you're also trying to conceive. In this chapter, we are going to take a look beyond the typical "diet and exercise" advice that is given by doctors or by well-meaning friends. It is time to learn the truth about weight loss and getting healthy. By following this plan, you can make a significant impact on your ability to conceive.

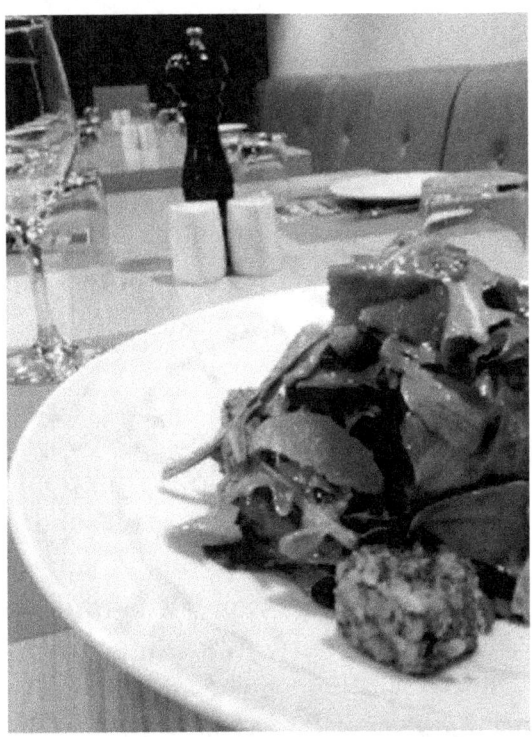

Taking a Look at the Proper Diet

When it comes to diet options today, we certainly are not lacking in possibilities. A simple look in the diet food aisle at your local grocery store will show you that you have many choices, including Weight Watchers, Jenny Craig, Atkins and other big names. When you take a look at what these weight loss companies have to offer, you see that they are approaching the subject from a variety of angles. Some reduce or raise carbohydrates, while others limit calories. Yet another option is low-fat, one that is often done improperly and unsuccessfully.

If you want to lose weight and to do so in the healthiest way possible, you need to base the majority of your diet on healthy starches. This would include food items such as rice, corn and potatoes. Approximately 40 to 50% of your plate should be starch, which is fairly easy for most people to do. The rest of the plate should be a combination of vegetables, along with very little meat, if any at all. Although the healthiest option would be to eat a vegan diet and to avoid meat, it is not something that most people are able to do, so it is not something that I recommend. Try to limit the amount of meat that you are eating, however, because it can impact your health.

One other piece of advice that I can give you for eating this type of diet is to avoid any type of oil. This would include so-called "healthy oils", such as olive oil and coconut oil. According to studies that were done on individuals with type II diabetes, their sugar problems went away when they ate a diet that was 70% table sugar and 30% white rice. When oil was reintroduced into the diet, however, they began to have problems with diabetes again. Avoid oil in your diet as much as possible and it may help your health significantly.

Why Should You Exercise?

Another option for being as healthy as possible is to get exercise. Exercising on a regular basis, including a healthy combination of cardiovascular and weight-bearing exercises can have a significant impact on your overall health and your ability to conceive. It will affect your entire body in a positive way, including improving your cardiovascular system and giving you more stamina. It is what takes place behind the scenes, however, that can really affect your ability to get pregnant.

As we discussed in a previous chapter, there is a delicate balance of hormones that is associated with your monthly cycle. This would include hormones that cause your body to make an egg mature and release it and other hormones, such as estrogen and progesterone, which cause the lining of your uterus to build up and then to shed. Unfortunately, many women have an imbalance of hormones and it can cause significant problems.

Exercising on a regular basis, even if you don't lose weight as a result of it, will likely improve your odds of conception. In fact, there were many women that were not able to ovulate who started ovulating after they begin exercising. It can also help to balance out your hormone levels and can have a significant impact on your overall health, even outside of the possibility of conception.

How Much Is Too Much?

Most people begin to cringe at this point, feeling as if they need to maintain a lean, tight body in order to conceive. Although it may be preferable for the way that you feel about yourself, it is not typically necessary for you to lose that much body fat in order to begin to see the benefits. In fact, with a moderate amount of weight loss of approximately 10%, you will likely begin to experience the benefits, which includes increasing the odds that you will conceive.

Beyond Diet and Exercise

Although diet and exercise are important for improving your odds of conceiving, they are not the only option that is available. You should also consider the other healthy lifestyle choices, including getting plenty of sleep every night, drinking lots of water and avoiding stress when possible. When you are able to do so, you may find that it is not only possible to get pregnant, it becomes relatively easy.

8. For Her: Getting the Right Fluids

In the previous chapter, we discussed the importance of remaining healthy if you want to increase your odds of conceiving a child. That would include eating a proper diet, losing weight if you are obese and getting some exercise. Another factor that you need to consider, however, is the fluids that you are taking in on a daily basis. In this chapter, we are going to consider a few different options and why you may want to make some changes now rather than waiting until later.

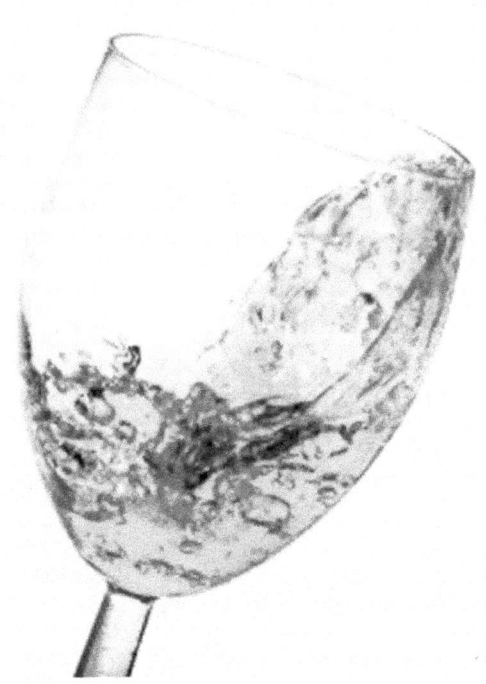

First of all, it's important to recognize that many people are dealing with a problem with chronic dehydration. As a matter of fact, they may have been dehydrated for the majority of their lives, and it certainly can have an impact on their health. If you are trying to conceive, it is best if you remain hydrated because that allows your body to work as fluidly as possible. It may even help to balance out your hormones, which can be a problem that would cause you to be unable to conceive as well.

There are also many alternative drinks that people like to consume, including sports drinks, coffee and alcohol. Although this book is not about quitting all of those items and it certainly is not going to tell you that it is wrong to drink on occasion or to have a cup of coffee every day, you may want to consider your overall health when it comes to conceiving a child. This chapter is going to take a look at the types of fluid that you should be drinking and what you may need to avoid if you want to improve your odds of becoming pregnant.

Alcohol - Obviously, if you are pregnant, you would want to avoid drinking alcohol because drinking too much could be harmful to the unborn child. It is best to avoid alcohol altogether during the time that you are pregnant but some women do have an occasional drink, such as a small glass of wine one or two times per week. As long as you are not getting drunk, the effect on the unborn child is going to be minimal.

Of course, drinking too much alcohol can have a negative effect on both you and the child. If you're trying to conceive a child, and you are successful in doing so, you're not going to be aware of the fact that you are pregnant for quite some time. If you are regularly consuming alcohol during that time, it can have an effect on the unborn child at a very early stage in your pregnancy.

You also need to consider the effect of alcohol before you become pregnant. If you drink alcohol on a regular basis and you consume too much alcohol, it can impact your ability to conceive a child. There are some studies that show that it can decrease fertility in women and if you drink excessively, including 10 drinks or more per week; it can have an even further impact on your ability to conceive. Although having a glass of wine or a drink every now and again is not going to have a significant impact, you would want to avoid excessive alcohol usage if you are trying to get pregnant.

Caffeine - Another beverage that is commonly consumed on a daily basis is coffee and there are also many sodas and specialty drinks that contain a significant amount of caffeine as well. It is important to recognize that these caffeinated drinks are not only something that is enjoyed by many women; caffeine is a drug that many of us are addicted to.

There are not any significant studies that have shown that caffeine can affect conception, but there is at least one study that shows that it does. While it may not have a significant effect on a woman that is able to conceive easily, if you are already having a difficulty with conception, it may be something that you want to consider avoiding. That is especially true if you use tobacco or alcohol, as the combination of those drugs can certainly harm your ability to conceive.

Water - If you want to improve your odds of conception and to stay as healthy as possible, you will drink plenty of clean water every day. The amount of water will differ from one woman to another, but it is typically recommended that you have a minimum of eight glasses of water on a daily basis. If you want a more specific number to aim for, try to drink half of your body weight every day in ounces of water and if you exercise or sweat regularly, increase that amount slightly.

The body is primarily made up of water, so obviously, you would want to make sure that you were remaining hydrated at all times. It really seems like a small thing to drink water, but as many of you know, it can be difficult to do regularly. When you make it a regular part of your life, however, it can have an impact on your health and it may even help you to conceive more easily.

9. For Her: Acupuncture and Other Alternative Options

At some point or another, many women that are having a difficulty conceiving a child are going to turn to some form of alternative treatment. In many cases, it involves a natural form of healing that takes the place of something that was done in ancient Chinese culture. An example of this is acupuncture, but there are many other forms of natural healing that claim to be able to assist in improving your ability to conceive. In this chapter, we are going to take a look at a few of those alternative forms of treatment so that you can make an informed decision as to whether you should try them or not.

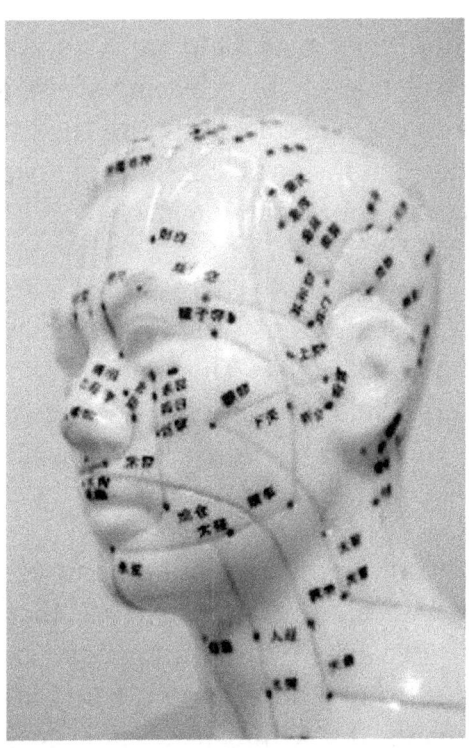

Acupuncture - This type of treatment has been around for thousands of years and it basically involves the insertion of tiny needles under the skin at various and specific points in the body. Primarily, this is done to improve the flow of energy that may have been pent up in some way or another. There are many people that have found success in using acupuncture for a variety of purposes, from weight loss and pain management to conception and successful childbirth. It may be something that you want to consider, as it is a harmless treatment that may be quite helpful.

Yoga - Another option that you may want to consider is the practice of yoga. This is also a practice that has its roots in ancient Chinese culture and many individuals have found it to be quite therapeutic, along with helpful for some very specific problems. When it comes to improving your odds of conception, using yoga may help in a number of different ways. Primarily, it does so by releasing stress and improving the blood flow in the body. In addition, the breathing that is associated with yoga may be able to help to lower your cortisol and can balance out your hormone levels.

Herbs and Vitamins - There are also a number of alternative therapy treatments that are associated with taking various herbs and vitamins. This is a very popular choice among many individuals, because it is easy to do and most of the items that you need to do it are inexpensive and readily available.

If you plan on using herbs and vitamins in order to improve your ability to conceive, it is important that you do your research in advance. There are a number of herbs, including those that come from roots, flowers, tree bark and extracts from various plants that claim to be able to help. Although they may be able to assist in this regard, you need to ensure that you are getting high quality products when you purchase them. Vitamins and herbs are not regulated by the FDA in the same way as prescription medications, so you need to do the footwork for yourself.

Deep Breathing Exercises - Along with yoga, which was mentioned above, you can also do various deep breathing exercises that may be able to assist to calm your nerves and to improve your ability to conceive. In fact, there are certain deep breathing exercises that are well known for their ability to calm the nerves and to balance out the oxygen and carbon dioxide levels in the body. One of those breathing exercises, known as square breathing, is even taught to first responders in an effort to help them to deal with very stressful situations that they may face on almost a daily basis.

These are only a few of the many different options that you have available. You might also appreciate trying options such as various types of massage, juice fasting and other forms of natural therapy. In some cases, they may make all the difference in your ability to conceive a child. Even if they don't help to improve your odds of conceiving, however, they're often very relaxing and certainly have that benefit associated with them as well.

10. For Couples: Frequency and Timing of Intercourse

One of the most common methods that are used worldwide for avoiding pregnancy is the rhythm method. This is a matter of timing intercourse in such a way that you would avoid the times when it was more likely for the woman to become pregnant. That time occurs approximately 14 days after the beginning of the menstrual cycle, which starts on the first day of your period. Many couples also use a similar method to try to conceive a child, working around that particular day and increasing the amount of intercourse that they have. Is this type of method truly effective?

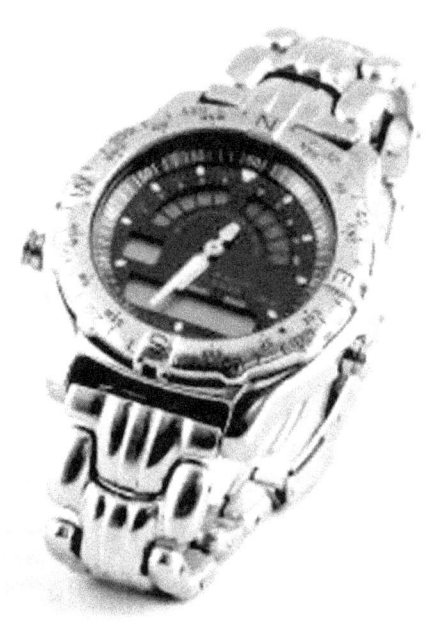

There are many different options that are available for timing your intercourse and increasing the frequency at the right times. It is important to understand, however, that any amount of intercourse is going to be ineffective if there is not an egg present. Unfortunately, it is very difficult, if not impossible to determine if that is the case, so it is important to continue to try and to work around the necessary time in order to effectively increase the odds of conception.

As far as the frequency of intercourse is concerned, this is often something that is misunderstood. As a matter of fact, there are two schools of thought that are associated with frequency that are both understood for different reasons.

Frequent Intercourse - Although statistically, couples that had intercourse every day did have a higher opportunity of conceiving a child, there may also be some problems with doing so. For one thing, it can be very stressful to have intercourse on a daily basis, and to try to maintain that level of intimacy and not to allow it to be done simply by rote. In addition, if you are having intercourse every day, the sperm production is not typically able to keep up with the timing. You may find that you are decreasing your odds of conceiving rather than improving it.

There is a frequency that does seem to work well, and that is having intercourse every other day. The sperm is able to live inside of the female body for anywhere from 3 to 5 days, so it is not necessary to have intercourse every day in order for the sperm to be present. If you have intercourse every other day, it gives the male the opportunity to produce new sperm effectively.

Storing It up - Another consideration that many couples try is avoiding intercourse for an extended amount of time in order to "store it up" and potentially, to increase the odds of conception. This is also a choice that does not tend to work well, but for the opposite reason as to why it does not work well if you have intercourse every day.

It is true that the amount of sperm that is produced is increased if you avoid intercourse for a certain amount of time but eventually, you're going to be working with the law of diminishing returns. In addition, after you go without intercourse for several days, the amount of unhealthy sperm that is available increases, so it actually decreases your ability to conceive. Stick with the intercourse every other day timing and you will increase your odds substantially.

Timing Intercourse Properly

It is also important for you to get the timing right, and this is one of the more difficult aspects because there is not really any significant sign as to when the woman ovulates. Some women claim to feel a slight pinch at the time of ovulation but for most women, it occurs without any noticeable effect. There is a way for you to determine when a woman ovulates, however, but it is going to take some work on your part.

For the most part, a woman is going to ovulate on or about the 14th day after the start of her menstrual cycle. That day may fluctuate by several days, depending upon her particular cycle and her chemical makeup. That being said, you can start with day 14 as a general point to begin testing to see when ovulation takes place.

Being able to identify the particular window of fertility, which may actually be quite small, is one of the most important factors to improving your odds of conception. When everything works as it should, the sperm is going to be able to live inside of the female body for up to five days and the egg that is released from the ovary will be available for one day during the time that it is traveling down the fallopian tubes. In essence, this gives a six-day window of fertility, but it is important for you to narrow things down more specifically if you are having difficulty conceiving.

During the time that a woman ovulates, her temperature is going to rise slightly. Constantly taking and checking the temperature of the woman is one of the only ways for you to fully determine when the window of fertility is at its peak. This can be a particular challenge, because it doesn't always happen during the time that the woman is awake. You can begin to check for the window fertility in advance, however, because it typically occurs at about the same time in your monthly cycle each and every month.

Modern medical science has also improved your odds of becoming pregnant by providing what is known as an ovulation prediction kit. These kits detect the rise of luteinizing hormone, which is associated with the release of the egg into the fallopian tubes. You may want to use one of these test kits along with checking your temperature frequently to determine when the best time is for you to become pregnant. You can then take advantage of it by timing intercourse according to that schedule.

11. For Couples: Kick the Habit

If someone were to tell you that smoking cigarettes was bad for your health, you would probably laugh at them. After all, it is something that all of us are aware of and the fact that smoking is bad for you is even printed on the side of each and every pack that you purchase. Included among the risks that are associated with smoking are heart disease, cancer, COPD and the list goes on and on. As far as it affecting your ability to conceive, you can also add that to the list as well.

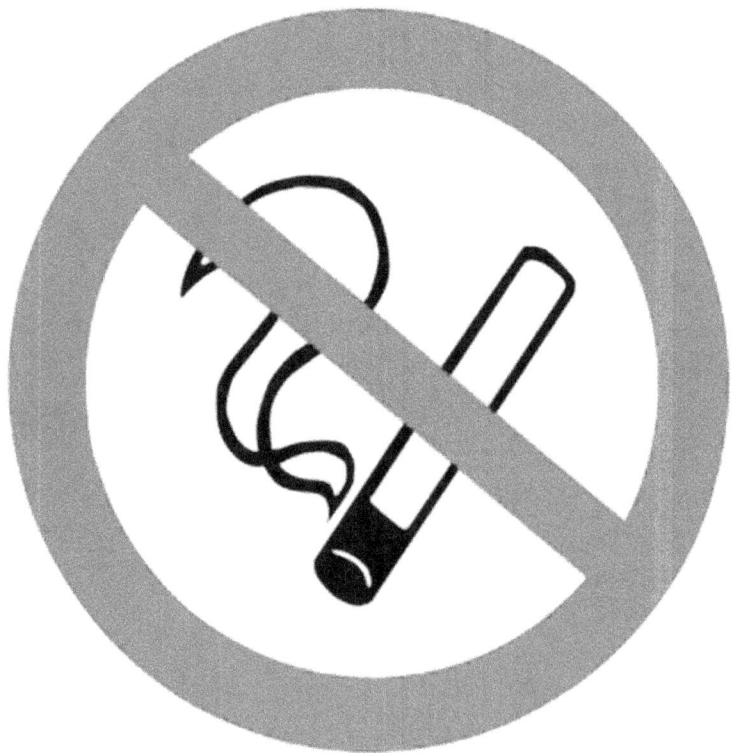

First of all, it is important to recognize that smoking during the time that you are pregnant, even in the early stages, can have a detrimental effect on the child. As we stated earlier in this publication on the subject of drinking alcohol, it is difficult to know when you're pregnant and you may go a month or two after conception before you recognize that you were successful. During that time, you may be affecting the health of the fetus by smoking cigarettes, and that is something that should be kept in mind as well.

What you may not recognize, however, is the fact that smoking cigarettes can actually affect your ability to get pregnant in the first place. It is estimated that many women who are over the age of 18 and who smoke cigarettes are dealing with some level of infertility, even if it is only minimal. If you are already having a difficulty with conceiving a child and you're also smoking cigarettes, you would be surprised to learn exactly how it is affecting your ability to conceive.

One of the ways in which smoking may affect conception is by affecting the egg before it ever leaves the follicle. There are a number of studies that show that the follicle itself may become damaged as a result of oxidative stress and may even cause DNA damage, resulting in certain levels of infertility. In addition, it may make changes to your cervix, to the fallopian tubes and can make it difficult for you to conceive a child or to carry a child to full term.

Although this publication is primarily based on the subject of being able to conceive a child, it is also important to recognize that infertility may also be associated with the inability to carry a child to term or to give birth to a live child. Cigarette smoking is not only associated with the inability to conceive a child, it can also increase the likelihood that you will have a miscarriage and can increase the odds of an ectopic pregnancy, which is not only devastating to the unborn child, it is very dangerous to the mother as well.

The best option that you have in front of you is to quit smoking, regardless of how much you smoke. In fact, even smoking half a pack of cigarettes a day may cause these difficulties. In addition, smoking may also affect the ability of the man to produce the sperm necessary to conceive a child, so there is a reason for you to approach the subject together. If the man smokes and the woman doesn't smoke, the secondary smoke that she is exposed to may cause such problems as well.

There are a number of options available for quitting smoking, but some of them may not be appropriate for a woman that is trying to conceive. It is important for you discuss the options with your physician and to decide on a treatment program that is going to work for both of you so that you can quit smoking permanently. More than likely, it will include some sort of therapy, typically in a group setting with other individuals that are trying to quit smoking as well.

It can be difficult to kick the habit but if you really want to improve your odds of conceiving a child, it will be well worth the journey. In addition, the increase in your overall health and the other benefits that giving up the habit provides will be worth the effort.

12. For Couples: Staying Healthy Together

In various chapters of this publication, we discussed options for building up your overall health in order to increase your odds of conceiving a child. Not only can it be beneficial for the man to increase his health, the fact is that both the man and woman can benefit from doing so.

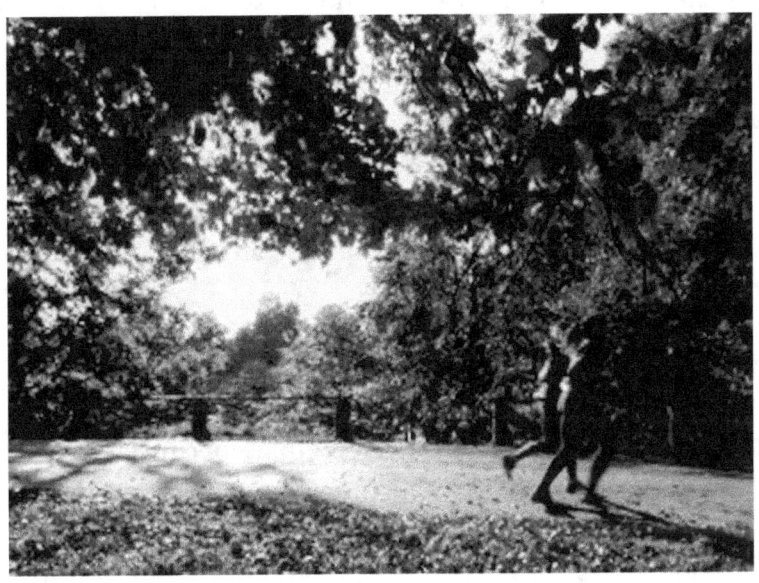

Unfortunately, the diet and exercise that is necessary for improving your health is often difficult to maintain for the long-term. That is why many couples have turned to helping each other in order to stick with the program and to make sure that they were able to improve their health in a way that would improve their odds of conception.

In addition, it can be very difficult for a couple when they are unable to conceive successfully for an extended amount of time. The intimacy that they may have shared together at one time has now become somewhat of a routine, as they are trying to time everything perfectly in order to have a child. The stress that is associated with infertility is also something that needs to be considered and, even though the couple was trying to produce something beautiful together, it may cause them to grow apart.

Often, it is beneficial for one person in the relationship to take the lead in making sure that both of them are as healthy as possible. Whenever the two of them are first starting out on any type of diet or exercise program, it is likely that one of them is going to want to quit before the other. It is true, however, that two people are able to stand together in a much more effective way than one person is able to stand apart from the other. If you work together to ensure that you stick with the diet and exercise program for the long-term, you will find that you are more successful at it.

In addition, it can be very strengthening to the relationship if you work toward a common goal such as this. Unfortunately, we tend to spend much of our lives apart because of work and other responsibilities that keep us from truly spending the time that we would like with each other. Going for a simple walk after you eat a good meal or perhaps taking the time to cook together in the kitchen and prepare your food expertly is going to help you to grow together as a couple and to make you more intimate with each other during this difficult time.

Although exercising together and eating a healthy diet is not a magic bullet, it certainly can be beneficial. It is something that you may want to consider, not only for the benefits that it provides in helping you to conceive but because it can help you to be a stronger couple and to stay together for the rest of your lives.

13. For Couples: Let Go of the Stress

Although there are many problems that couples may experience that can result in a decrease in their ability to conceive, stress is perhaps one of the leading problems in today's world. Unfortunately, many of us are dealing with levels of stress that are actually chronic, and we may find that we are never able to truly come down from our stress and all of the problems that are associated with it. An inability to conceive a child is one issue that you may find goes hand-in-hand with high levels of stress.

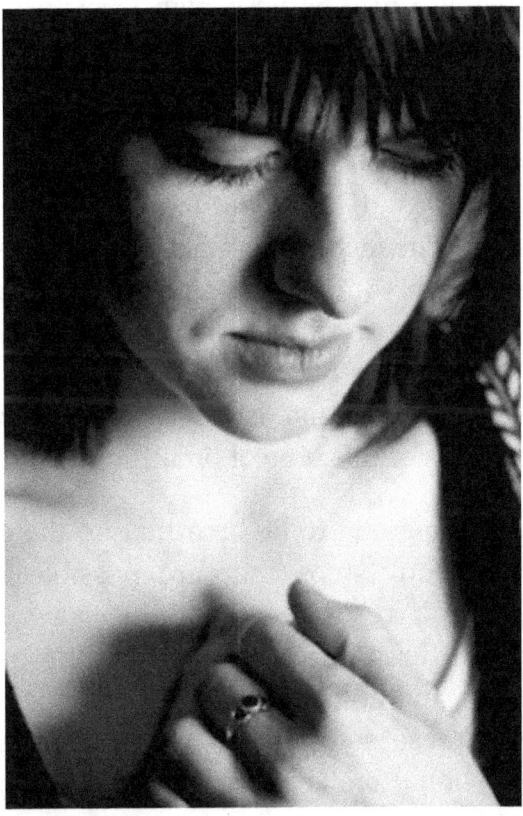

First of all, stress produces stress hormones, such as cortisol, and that can certainly have a significant impact on your overall hormone levels. As was discussed in a previous chapter in this publication, it is necessary for you to have a balance of hormones if you want to conceive successfully. During the time that a woman is going through her monthly cycle, increases and decreases in hormones such as estrogen, progesterone and follicle stimulating hormone are experienced. If any one of these hormones is at an imbalance, it can cause problems.

In addition, stress can also affect your overall health and that will have an impact on your ability to conceive a child as well. Many individuals struggle with their level of health, regardless of whether they are dealing with high levels of stress or not. When you struggle in such a way, it can certainly have an impact on your ability to conceive a child and to carry that child through to maturity and delivery.

Overcoming stress can be difficult, but it is certainly not going to be impossible. The fact of the matter is that there are many opportunities to overcome stress, including some that can be accomplished in a short amount of time and regularly, if you do it properly. This type of stress relief is available through a deep breathing exercise that is known as square breathing. What are the basics of this type of breathing exercise?

In essence, you are going to be breathing to the count of four for each of the four steps that are possible through this exercise. The first part is to breathe in through your nose, then you will hold your breath for the count of four, breathe out to the count of four and hold your lungs empty for the final four count. Each of these steps is not more important than the other and you should make sure that you follow them closely and pay attention to what is being done.

Square breathing can quickly balance the carbon dioxide and oxygen in your body. It is a process that is taught to first responders and it can certainly have the benefit of helping you to deal with stress in the greatest way possible. Although it is only a single option that is available for dealing with stress, it is certainly one that you should consider. When you are able to deal with stress successfully, you can deal with your overall health and may improve your ability to conceive.

14. For Couples: Is It Time to See a Doctor?

Throughout the pages of this publication, we have discussed many different options that may allow you to improve your ability to conceive a child successfully. For the most part, they were natural options and did not involve medical science in order to achieve the purpose. There may be times, however, when experiencing a problem with infertility may cause you to consider the possibility of talking to a higher authority. In this chapter, we're going to discuss the possibility of seeking attention through a medical professional.

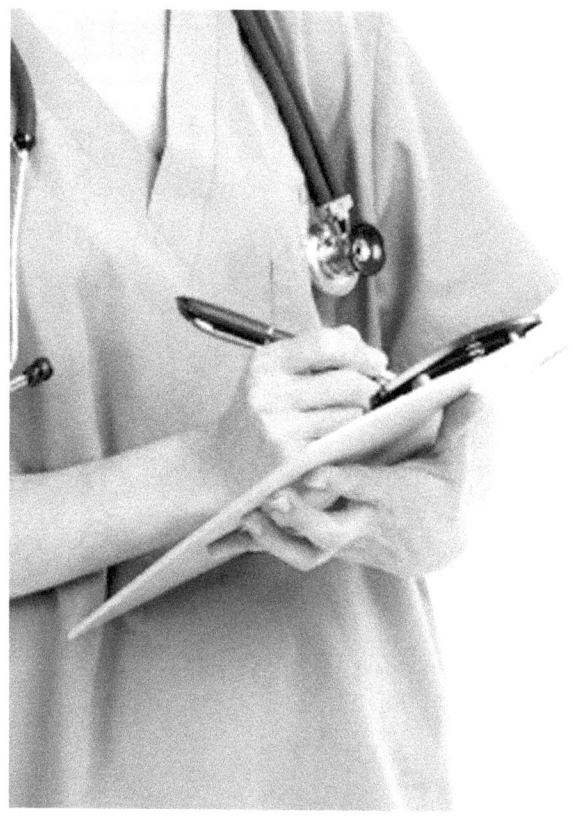

Fortunately, medical science has come a long way in the past decade or so in helping individuals who are unable to conceive successfully. Some of the options that may be discussed with you by your physician include the possibility of in vitro fertilization or perhaps taking a drug that would cause you to release eggs from the follicles.

In either case, it is improving your odds of conception but it may also be possible that it makes it difficult to conceive, or it may cause problems if conception does occur. For example, some of the fertility drugs that are on the market make it more likely for multiple eggs to be released from the ovaries. If there are multiple eggs available for fertilization, it may be possible that you will be carrying multiple babies as a result.

In vitro fertilization has also come a long way and it is a far cry from the options that were available not that long ago. In fact, you may be able to produce a number of fertile eggs and they can even be graded according to the possibility of successfully implanting themselves into the womb and providing you with a child. Of course, there are also some concerns along the way and these are things that will need to be discussed with your physician in advance of any pregnancy help being provided.

Modern medical science can certainly make a difference in your ability to conceive and carry a child through delivery. When you make the right decision and choose modern medical science along with other options that may be available, you will find that it is much easier for you to be successful in the conception of your child.

www.ingramcontent.com/pod-product-compliance
Lightning Source LLC
Chambersburg PA
CBHW070342290526
45791CB00003B/1437